Hodgkin Lymphoma:
Fast Focus Study Guide

JT Thomas, MD

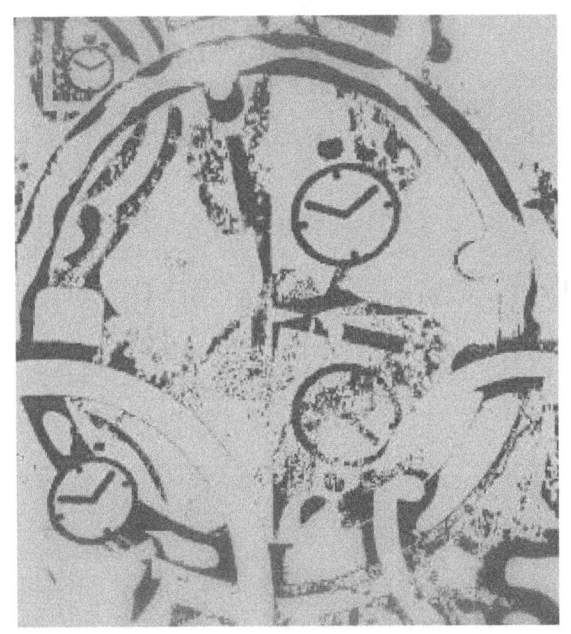

Acknowledgements

I dedicate this book to my beautiful wife and children, who I love more than all the water in all the oceans and all the seas.

CONTENTS

- This book is written to help the reader further understand Hodgkin Lymphoma.

- This book is written in a simple and easy to read format designed for medical students, residents and physicians who are preparing for boards.

- This book simplifies a complicated medical issue so you will remember the important details.

- You will not get caught up in the minutia. Just the facts are found in this book.

- This Fast Focus Study Guide will provide you with a practical review of the key information you need to know.

- Buy this book now if you want this quick and concise information

Hodgkin Lymphoma is a common lymphoma with a relatively good prognosis characterized by a clonal expansion of the B cells associated with the Reed-Sternberg cell first described in 1832 by Dr. Thomas Hodgkin.

Hodgkin lymphoma can be separated into Classical Hodgkin lymphoma and Nodular lymphocyte predominant Hodgkin lymphoma (NLPHL).

Classical Hodgkin lymphoma accounts for 95% of Hodgkin disease and is characterized by the Reed-Sternberg cells. Nodular lymphocyte predominant Hodgkin lymphoma accounts for 5% of Hodgkin disease and are characterized by variants of Reed-Sternberg cells called popcorn cells.

Reed-Sternberg cells express the lymphocyte-associated marker CD30. These cells do not consistently stain with markers for B or T cells. Molecular techniques using single Reed-Sternberg cells show that there is clonal immunoglobulin gene rearrangements present. It has been determined that Reed-Sternberg cells are of B-cell origin.

Classic Hodgkin lymphoma has 4 subtypes: Nodular sclerosis Hodgkin disease, mixed cellularity Hodgkin disease, lymphocyte-rich Hodgkin disease, and lymphocyte-depleted Hodgkin disease.

Nodular sclerosis is the commonest histological subtype and is characterized by bands of fibrosis that enclose nodules of lymphoid tissue containing variable numbers of Hodgkin cells.

Mixed cellularity Hodgkin lymphoma is characterized by the presence of a heterogeneous mixture of lymphocytes, eosinophils, neutrophils, plasma cells, epithelial cells and Hodgkin's cells. In general, the more lymphocytes present, the fewer the number of Hodgkin cells and the better the prognosis.

Mixed cellularity Hodgkin's lymphoma has an unfavorable prognosis.

Lymphocyte-predominant Hodgkin lymphoma does not have a bimodal distribution and has a median age at diagnosis of 35 years old.

Lymphocyte-predominant Hodgkin lymphoma accounts for approximately 5% of Hodgkin's lymphoma.

Lymphocyte predominant Hodgkin lymphoma is CD20 positive, CD30 negative, and CD 15 negative.

Lymphocyte-depleted Hodgkin lymphoma has the worst prognosis.

Approximately 70% of patients with Hodgkin lymphoma have an enlarged non-tender lymph node in the neck.

The spleen and para aortic lymph nodes are involved in 34% of patients with Hodgkin's lymphoma.

In stage I Hodgkin lymphoma only 1 lymph node area or lymphoid organ such as the thymus is involved. If the cancer is found only in 1 area of a single organ outside of the lymph system it is termed stage IE (extralymphatic).

In stage II disease the lymphoma is in 2 or more groups of lymph nodes on the same side of the diaphragm. If the lymphoma extends from these lymph node(s) into an organ it is termed stage IIE.

In stage III disease the lymphoma involves lymph node areas on both sides of the diaphragm. If the lymphoma involves an area or organ next to the lymph nodes it is termed IIIE. If it spreads into the spleen it is staged IIIS. If it involves both the spleen and the extra lymphatic area it is stage IIISE.

Hodgkin lymphoma is stage IV if it has spread outside the lymph system into an organ that is not right next to an involved node. Lymphoma that involves the bone marrow, liver, brain or spinal cord, or the pleura is stage IV.

The letter B is added to the stage if the patient experiences B symptoms such as loss of more than 10% of body weight over the previous 6 months (without dieting), unexplained fever of at least 101.5°F, or drenching night sweats.

The letter X is added to the stage if the tumors in the chest that are at least one-third as wide as the chest, or tumors in other areas are at least 10 centimeters across.

Stage I or II is considered early stage. The first objective when someone has stage I or II is to define favorable or unfavorable.

Unfavorable factors for stage I-II Hodgkin
disease include

-ESR> 50

-Mediastinal mass >1/3 the total thorax
(Treated Different)

-Any B symptoms

-> 3 nodal sites

-Any lymph node mass > 10 cm (Bulky)

If the patient has stage I or II disease and does not have any of the unfavorable factors listed on the previous page then they are considered early stage favorable.

The treatment for early stage favorable is based on the HD 10 trial. The treatment is ABVD x 2 cycles followed by 20 gy radiation.

The treatment for early stage unfavorable without bulky disease is based on the HD 11 trial. The treatment is ABVD x 4 cycles followed by 30 Gy radiation.

The treatment for early stage unfavorable with bulky disease ($\geq$10 cm) is ABVD x 6 cycles followed by involved field radiation to 36 gy.

Treatment for stage III and IV disease is dependent on risk factors as demonstrated by the Hodgkin Lymphoma International Prognostic Score.

The International Prognostic Index with a prognostic score that is based on following seven adverse factors

Albumin level of <4.0 g/dL.

Hemoglobin level of <10.5 g/dL.

Male sex.

Age of $\geq$45 years.

Stage IV disease.

White blood cell (WBC) count of $\geq$15,000/mm3.

Absolute lymphocytic count of <600/mm3 or a lymphocyte count that was <8% of the total WBC count.

Patients with stage III or stage IV Hodgkin lymphoma with 4 or more risk factors should receive 6 cycles of escalated BEACOPP.

The treatment for relapsed or refractory

Hodgkin lymphoma is somewhat

different.

The first thing is to repeat the biopsy, staging, assessment of adverse factors.

It is important to get the patient to autologous stem cell transplant. One approach is 2 cycles of ICE chemotherapy followed by stem cell harvest and PET scan. If PET is negative take to high dose chemotherapy and stem cell transplant. If PET is positive then proceed with gemcitabine, vinorelbine, doxorubicin x 4 cycles. If PET negative at that time, take to high dose chemotherapy and stem cell transplant.

A negative PET scan prior to transplant is an important prognostic indicator.

Autologous stem cell transplant (ASCT) in patients with relapsed or refractory Hodgkin lymphoma can achieve cure in approximately 50% of patients.

Brentuximab vedotin is given to try to prevent relapse after autologous stem cell transplant. Brentuximab vedotin is a CD30 directed therapy that has shown efficacy in patients with Hodgkin lymphoma who relapsed or were refractory after prior autologous stem cell transplant.

Early consolidation post autologous stem cell transplant with Brentuximab vedotin demonstrated improved PFS survival.

The most common side effect of Brentuximab

is neuropathy.

Brentuximab cannot be combined with gemcitabine or bleomycin because of pulmonary toxicity.

There are other options on the horizon. Pembrolizumab is a humanized monoclonal IgG4 antibody against PD-1 that has shown activity in patients with relapsed or refractory Hodgkin disease.

Pembrolizumab showed activity in patients in this situation. The drug showed a 21% complete remission rate and a 66% ORR. This medication was associated with an 86% clinical benefit rate.

This concludes Hodgkin Lymphoma: Fast Focus Study Guide

Search Amazon Kindle books to find other study guides written by

JT Thomas, MD

Internal Medicine Study Guide

Hematology Study Guide

Medical Oncology Study Guide

Cardiology Study Guide

Multiple Myeloma Study Guide

Differential Diagnosis Study Guide

Rheumatology Study Guide

Cancer Study Guide